Make Your Home Free of Toxic Chemicals

Introduction

Nobody wants *toxic chemicals* in their home. However, many people have *toxic chemicals* in their home, yet they are unaware that those dangers are lurking there.

We live in a culture where *toxic chemicals* are just a part of life. Or so it sometimes seems. And they just seem to creep into our homes.

Dale Stubbart

Author of <u>Traveling with Multiple Chemical Sensitivities</u>

Make Your Home Free of *Toxic Chemicals*

Once those *toxic chemicals* are in our homes, it may seem daunting, almost impossible, to get them out of our homes. We try everything, short of exorcism to rid them from our homes. Sometimes nothing seems to work.

Over thirty years of attempts, failures, and successes at ridding our homes of *toxic chemicals* have led to the creation of this plan. It takes a lot of work. And you will no doubt be overwhelmed by it at first glance.

Dale Stubbart

Author of <u>Traveling with Multiple Chemical Sensitivities</u>

Make Your Home Free of Toxic Chemicals

But the plan does work. And the end results are worth both the time and the effort. Removing *toxic chemicals* from a home, often results in the inhabitants being better able to breathe easier, being sick less often, and having more energy.

It takes time. But it can be accomplished step by step. Do as much as you can. And do what works for you. Then move on to the next step.

You may need to come back to the first steps and perform the remaining tasks. But eventually, you will work out

Author of <u>Traveling with Multiple Chemical Sensitivities</u>

Make Your Home Free of Toxic Chemicals

what works for you. You will work out what rids your home from *toxic chemicals* to the point, that you can live at peace with your home again.

Dale Stubbart

Author of <u>Traveling with Multiple Chemical Sensitivities</u>

Make Your Home Free

of Toxic Chemicals

Table of Contents

Author of <u>Traveling with Multiple Chemical Sensitivities</u>

Make Your Home Free of Toxic Chemicals

Author of <u>Traveling with Multiple Chemical Sensitivities</u>

Make Your Home Free of Toxic Chemicals

Make Your Home Free of Toxic Chemicals

Author of <u>Traveling with Multiple Chemical Sensitivities</u>

Make Your Home Free of Toxic Chemicals

Author of <u>Traveling with Multiple Chemical Sensitivities</u>

Make Your Home Free of Toxic Chemicals

Author of <u>Traveling with Multiple Chemical Sensitivities</u>

Make Your Home Free *of Toxic Chemicals*

Make Your Home Free of Toxic Chemicals

What Makes a Chemical Toxic?

There are many, various *toxic chemicals*. The most prevalent *toxic chemicals* are carbon–based. But why are these chemicals *toxic*?

These chemicals are derived from Petroleum and are called Petrochemicals. Petroleum or oil comes from the days of the dinosaurs. And perhaps if you had to travel all the way through a dinosaur's digestive tract you might be toxic too.

Dale Stubbart

Author of <u>Traveling with Multiple Chemical Sensitivities</u>

Make Your Home Free of Toxic Chemicals

But seriously, chemicals are *toxic* based on their structure, the rate at which we absorb them, and our ability to eliminate them or to turn them into a non–toxic or less toxic substance.

Toxicity can cause damage to an organ, disrupt a biological process, or disturb an enzyme system.

Petrochemicals are found in gasoline, kerosene, plastic, acrylics, polyester, nylon, spandex, etc. Petrochemicals are often found in fragrances, soaps,

Make Your Home Free of Toxic Chemicals

detergents, solvents, paints, drugs, fertilizer, pesticides, tires, and insulation.

If I understand it correctly, Petrochemicals cause us to have less tolerance for other stress factors. Petrochemicals become even more *toxic* when they are extracted, because they are combined with Chlorine at that time. And Chlorine is another very *toxic* and very prevalent chemical.

Petrochemicals also contain Sulfur which can become *toxic* when mixed with other substances. Sulfuric acid, for instance is very corrosive.

Dale Stubbart
Author of <u>Traveling with Multiple Chemical Sensitivities</u>

Make Your Home Free
of Toxic Chemicals

I suspect that refined crude oil is more *toxic* than unrefined crude oil. My suspicion is based on the extra chemicals which are added in the refining process. It doesn't really matter though, because crude oil is *toxic* whether it is refined or not.

The side effects of Petrochemicals may include shortness of breath, eye irritation, dizziness, cough, nose congestion, sore throat, phlegm, and weakness.

Make Your Home Free of Toxic Chemicals

https://www.ncbi.nlm.nih.gov/pubmed/24851575

Many other highly *toxic chemicals* contain Lead, Mercury, or Fluoride.

Chlorine prevents bacteria from growing. It also interferes with our breathing. You will find chlorine in bleach, pools, and in drinking water. Experts may say that low levels of chlorine are not *toxic*. I beg to differ.

The side effects of Chlorine may include airway irritation, wheezing,

Author of <u>Traveling with Multiple Chemical Sensitivities</u>

Make Your Home Free of Toxic Chemicals

having a difficult time breathing, sore throat, cough, chest tightness, eye irritation, and skin irritation. Chlorine gas was used to kill people in Nazi concentration camps.
https://www.health.ny.gov/environmental/emergency/chemical_terrorism/chlorine_general.htm

At low levels, sulfur itself may not be *toxic*, unless you're allergic to it. But sulfur is often combined with other things which make it *toxic*.

Author of <u>Traveling with Multiple Chemical Sensitivities</u>

Make Your Home Free of Toxic Chemicals

The side effects of Sulfur may include burning, stinging, tingling, itching, redness, dryness, peeling, and irritation. https://www.everydayhealth.com/drugs/sulfur-topical

Lead is not often found in the US, other than in very old paint and very old pipes. Lead gets distributed throughout your body in much the same way as beneficial minerals. This is similar to how other *toxic* heavy metals accumulate in our bodies.

Make Your Home Free of Toxic Chemicals

The side effects of lead may include developmental delay, learning difficulties, irritability, loss of appetite, weight loss, sluggishness and fatigue, abdominal pain, vomiting, constipation, hearing loss, seizures, and eating things such as paint chips which aren't food (pica).
https://www.mayoclinic.org/diseases-conditions/lead-poisoning/symptoms-causes/syc-20354717

Mercury is another *toxic* heavy metal. Mercury can be lurking in old thermometers, fluorescent and compact

Author of <u>Traveling with Multiple Chemical Sensitivities</u>

Make Your Home Free of Toxic Chemicals

fluorescent (CFL) bulbs, tanning lamps, and batteries.

The side effects of mercury may include mood swings, nervousness, irritability, other emotional changes, insomnia, headaches, abnormal sensations, muscle twitching, tremors, weakness, muscle atrophy, decreased cognitive functions, kidney malfunction, respiratory failure, and death. https://www.emedicinehealth.com/mercury_poisoning/article_em.htm#what_are_the_symptoms_of_mercury_poisoning

Author of <u>Traveling with Multiple Chemical Sensitivities</u>

Make Your Home Free of Toxic Chemicals

Cadmium is another *toxic* heavy metal. Cadmium may be present around mining activities. Cadmium might be found in fertilizer, batteries, pigments, and plastic.

Side effects of cadmium may include food poisoning symptoms, bronchitis, pneumonitis, pulmonary edema (too much fluid in the lungs), hyperemia (too much blood in the blood vessels), thrombosis (blood clots), nausea, vomiting, and diarrhea.

https://www.atsdr.cdc.gov/csem/csem.asp?csem=6&po=11

Make Your Home Free of Toxic Chemicals

Other *toxic* heavy metals include Arsenic, Chromium, Thallium, and Antimony.
https://www.lenntech.com/processes/heavy/heavy-metals/heavy-metals.htm

Now that I've totally ruined your day, just keep in mind that there are a lot of *toxic chemicals* out there. Focus on eliminating those which you are most susceptible to and which you are most likely to encounter.

For most people these would be Petrochemicals, Cadmium, and Mercury.

Dale Stubbart

Page **22** of **140**

Author of <u>Traveling with Multiple Chemical Sensitivities</u>

Make Your Home Free

of *Toxic Chemicals*

I would also focus on eliminating
Chlorine and *Toxic Mold.*

Author of <u>Traveling with Multiple
Chemical Sensitivities</u>

Make Your Home Free of Toxic Chemicals

Multiple Chemical Sensitivities

It is estimated that one in five people living in the US are affected by Multiple Chemical Sensitivities (MCS). Most people with MCS, however, are unaware that they have these sensitivities.

People with MCS may be aware that they have these sensitivities and think that it is just part of normal life. They usually don't know that there is a clinical term for them.

Make Your Home Free of Toxic Chemicals

If you have MCS, it basically means that you are very sensitive to a variety of chemicals.

MCS is also called Idiopathic Environmental Intolerances (IEI) or just Environmental Intolerance (EI).

My wife is very sensitive to every man-made chemical. There may be a few exceptions, but none that we have come across. The common ingredient in these chemicals is Petroleum.

Make Your Home Free of Toxic Chemicals

These man-made chemicals cause her severe face pain and brain fog. They deplete her energy.

In order to live a decent life and not be bombarded constantly by these chemicals, we have had to change our lifestyle. *Toxic chemicals* have become the bane of our existence. We have had to remove them from our homes.

In this book, I will share with you a plan that we have developed over thirty years, while living in five different homes

Dale Stubbart

Author of <u>Traveling with Multiple Chemical Sensitivities</u>

Make Your Home Free of Toxic Chemicals

and remedying them of their infestation of *toxic chemicals*.

I was originally going to title this book <u>Living with Multiple Chemical Sensitivities</u>. But I thought that I would expand the information a bit, in order to make it helpful to more people. I did so and retitled this book <u>Make Your Home Free of *Toxic Chemicals*</u>.

If you have MCS and want to travel more, please read my book, <u>Traveling</u>

Dale Stubbart

Author of <u>Traveling with Multiple Chemical Sensitivities</u>

Make Your Home Free of Toxic Chemicals

with <u>Multiple Chemical Sensitivities</u>.
Thanks.

<u>What Would Terry Do</u>, is my book of humorous stories about the constraints of living with this debilitating disease. And believe me, if you do have to live with this malady, you need to find reasons to laugh.

While this book is humorous, it also lists several resources for dealing with MCS. You might find it to be a companion book to this one.

Dale Stubbart

Author of <u>Traveling with Multiple Chemical Sensitivities</u>

Make Your Home Free of Toxic Chemicals

You can find resources for dealing with MCS on my website –
https://www.princesstigerlily.com/mcs

Make Your Home Free of Toxic Chemicals

The Plan to Remove Toxic Chemicals From Your Home

One way to remove *toxic chemicals* from your home is to try to identify everything which contains *toxic chemicals* and remove those items. That particular method might quickly overwhelm you.

Our approach removes *toxic chemicals* in stages. The most *toxic* ones are removed

Make Your Home Free of Toxic Chemicals

first. Our approach also cleans up the most important rooms first. Our plan starts with the bedroom since that's where you spend at least six to eight hours per day. At least we hope you get that much sleep.

Each stage of our plan includes both the items containing *toxic chemicals* to be removed during that stage and the rooms to be cleaned up during that stage. The items containing *toxic chemicals* to be removed, are to be remedied throughout the entire premises. The rooms we

Make Your Home Free of *Toxic Chemicals*

address at each stage need further attention with regards to *toxic chemicals*.

Here are the stages of the plan:

- **Stage One – Spring Green –** Eliminate the Most Prevalent Items with the Highest *Toxicity*
- **Stage Two – Chartreuse –** Eliminate Less Prevalent Items with the Highest *Toxicity*
- **Stage Three – Lime Green –** Clean up the Air, Water, and Light
- **Stage Four – Living Green –** Extra Air Purification

Make Your Home Free of Toxic Chemicals

- Stage Five – Avocado Green – Further Interior Remediation
- Stage Six – Forest Green – Exterior Remediation
- Stage Seven – Emerald Green – Further Exterior Remediation

As you work each stage of the plan, you may substitute other criteria than those listed, so long as the substitution satisfies the overall objective of that stage.

Make Your Home Free of *Toxic Chemicals*

As with every plan, do what makes sense for you and your situation. Also do what works for you.

Stage One is really important to complete. And it is really important to complete it first. Perform the other stages as it makes sense to you to complete them.

You may decide to stop at some point after Stage One and not complete the rest of the steps. That's ok. But if you really want to make your home free from *toxic chemicals*, you will want to

Make Your Home Free of Toxic Chemicals

complete most of the criteria in the first five stages.

Also, it's ok to take breaks. Complete what you can. Take a break. And then come back and complete some more steps. Not all of us have indispensable amounts of energy.

When you complete each stage, take some time to celebrate. Give yourself a pat on the back for this accomplishment. Treat completing each stage as a major breakthrough. You're on your way to a

Make Your Home Free of Toxic Chemicals

cleaner home, one which is free of *toxic chemicals*!

If seven stages seems overwhelming, complete Stage One. Then skip to the end of the book where you will find simpler plans.

Make Your Home Free
of Toxic Chemicals

Stage One – Spring Green – Eliminate the Most Prevalent Items With the Highest Toxicity

Intro

Stage One of our plan to rid your home of *toxic chemicals* suggests scoring 40 out of 40 points from the following 4 criterion (10 points for each). These are

Author of <u>Traveling with Multiple Chemical Sensitivities</u>

Make Your Home Free of Toxic Chemicals

the most important items to complete. And it is very important to totally complete them. Not to worry, completing them is not very difficult.

Stage One looks at those items which are most likely to make those living in your home sick. When we remove these items, the residents of your home have a better chance of recovering, not getting sick in the first place, having more energy, and feeling better to boot.

This is not a medical opinion. It is our lived experience.

Author of <u>Traveling with Multiple Chemical Sensitivities</u>

Make Your Home Free of Toxic Chemicals

Here is the list of items that you will want to eliminate or greatly reduce. If you think of others, go ahead and get rid of them also; so long as you don't get side-tracked from accomplishing this objective.

Remove All Air Fresheners

Remove all air fresheners, especially plug-in air fresheners from your home. And quit using them. You may want to post a list in your home of approved natural air fresheners. This list would perhaps include citric spritzes, vodka,

Make Your Home Free of Toxic Chemicals

etc. The items on this list would be those with no fragrances and those with only very light natural fragrances.

Switch to Natural Laundry Products

This includes:

- Not using Chlorine.
- Not using chlorinated products.
- Using a natural, unscented laundry detergent. (The best ones are those which are safe for septic systems.)
- Or use baking soda and/or vinegar in place of natural laundry detergent.

Dale Stubbart   Page **40** of **140**
Author of <u>Traveling with Multiple Chemical Sensitivities</u>

Make Your Home Free of Toxic Chemicals

- Use natural fabric softener (or none).
- Use natural dryer sheets (or none).
- Use natural (non–Chlorine) bleach (or none).

Switch to Natural, Non-Toxic Personal-Care Products

These include:

- Soaps
- Shampoos, Conditioner, Mousse, etc.
- Deodorant, Antiperspirant, etc.
- Toothpaste, Mouthwash

Make Your Home Free of Toxic Chemicals

- Antibacterial wipes
- Lotions
- Sunscreen
- Lip balm
- Makeup
- Nail Polish
- Etc.

Do Not Allow Smoking

Make smoking not allowed in your home. You may want to post signs to indicate this.

Several states do not allow smoking in public buildings or within 15–20 feet or

Make Your Home Free of Toxic Chemicals

more of entrances (including windows) to those buildings. Although your home is a private building, you may want to consider similar rules or guidelines.

Cigarettes contain many *toxic chemicals.* They can cause cancer, heart disease, etc. Just read the label for that list of *side effects.*

Make Your Home Free of Toxic Chemicals

Rooms to Pay the Most Attention To

The room to pay the most attention to during this first stage is the room where you spend the most time. That would be your bedroom.

Most people spend six to eight hours in their bedroom every night. I would like to say that they sleep for that many hours. But many people have trouble sleeping.

Make Your Home Free of Toxic Chemicals

Most people spend much of the rest of their day outside of their house. The remaining time is often spent in the kitchen or dining room and in the living room or recreation room.

Even if you don't spend most of your time in your bedroom, you probably still go there to try to sleep and rejuvenate. Rejuvenation is more difficult to achieve when *toxic chemicals* are present. And even if you remove all the *toxic chemicals* from your bedroom, it does you little good, if you keep bringing them back in.

Author of <u>Traveling with Multiple Chemical Sensitivities</u>

Make Your Home Free of *Toxic Chemicals*

The bedrooms should be small areas. Ideally bedrooms contain the bed and not much else. This helps keep *toxic chemicals* out of the sleeping area. And that is important when you are trying to help your immune system recover from the *toxic chemicals* which it encounters in a normal day.

Other rooms to pay special attention to during this first phase are those rooms where you want to concentrate, study, meditate, etc. It's harder to keep your

Make Your Home Free

of Toxic Chemicals

mind focused when it's being inundated with *toxic chemicals*. Now what was I saying?

Make Your Home Free of Toxic Chemicals

Toxic Chemicals On Us

Often people carry *toxic chemicals* on their bodies. This happens in three ways.

One: People wear their shoes inside the house. These are the same shoes that they wore in the parking lot on the way to the store. These are the same shoes that they wore inside the store. These are the same shoes they wore when they walked across a pesticided lawn, etc.

Make Your Home Free of Toxic Chemicals

Take off your shoes when you come in and leave them by the door. Better yet, leave them outside if practical.

Two: People wear clothes which have laundry fragrances on them. Perhaps their clothes just picked up these fragrances while they were out and about.

Perhaps their clothes have been dried with a dryer-sheet. Even the non-fragranced commercial big brand ones contain perfume.

Make Your Home Free of Toxic Chemicals

Perhaps their clothes were washed with a scented laundry detergent.

Dale Stubbart
Author of <u>Traveling with Multiple Chemical Sensitivities</u>

Make Your Home Free of Toxic Chemicals

However it was that their clothes came by those fragrances, the fragrances most likely contain *toxic chemicals*.

Three: People's body and/or hair have picked up one or more personal fragrances. These fragrances may have come from

- Soap
- Shampoo
- Body Spray
- Perfume
- Cologne
- Deodorant

Make Your Home Free of Toxic Chemicals

- Etc.

All you would have to do is to walk by within ten feet of fragrances, and they're all over you. Yes, some of those fragrances are that strong. And yes, most of them contain *toxic chemicals*.

Once we pick up these fragrances and their accompanying or inherent *toxic chemicals*, they are hard to get rid of. So we just carry them around with us everywhere we go.

Make Your Home Free of Toxic Chemicals

Baking Soda, Vinegar, Tea Bags, and Vodka are some of the best odor removers there are when it comes to dealing with these *toxic chemicals.* Sometimes just being out in the weather helps.

You can read about how to get rid of fragrances in my book <u>Traveling with Multiple Chemical Sensitivities</u>. For now, just wash your clothes and take a shower.

Make Your Home Free of Toxic Chemicals

And whatever you do, don't get cleaned up and then put on fragrances which contain *toxic chemicals*.

That's it for Stage One. Simple enough, right?

Make Your Home Free
of Toxic Chemicals

Stage Two – Chartreuse – Eliminate Less Prevalent Items Which Are Also Very Toxic

Intro

Stage Two of our plan to rid your home of *toxic chemicals* suggests scoring 30 out of 50 points from the following 5

Make Your Home Free of Toxic Chemicals

criterion (10 points for each).
Completion of Stage Two means that
you have also completed Stage One.

Stage Two looks at more items which
are most likely to make those living in
your home sick. Stage Two used to be
part of Stage One. But there were just
too many items to make Stage One
manageable. That is especially true since
most people try to tackle Stage One right
after they move into a new home or
shortly after they learn that *toxic chemicals*
are making them less well than they
want to be.

Dale Stubbart

Author of <u>Traveling with Multiple
Chemical Sensitivities</u>

Make Your Home Free of Toxic Chemicals

Make Your Lawn Natural or Organic

- Switch to natural or organic lawn-care products.
- Remove chemical pesticides and herbicides from the premises.
- You may want to post a *Pesticide-Free* or *Salmon-Safe* or *No Spray* sign in your yard once you have switched to a toxic-free yard.

Switch to Natural, Non-Toxic Home Cleaning Products

Make Your Home Free of Toxic Chemicals

There are plenty of non-toxic alternatives available, though you may be able to find them easier on the internet than in your local grocery or home improvement store.

You'll also want to remove solvents from your home. Vinegar may work just as well for most if not all of what you were using solvents for.

Hire a Professional Mold Inspector

Hire a mold inspector who knows about natural mold remedies to inspect

Make Your Home Free of Toxic Chemicals

your home. Then employ their recommended methods for eliminating any mold and potential mold problems.

Remediate Asbestos

Make certain that any asbestos within your home is properly remediated. Probably all you will need to do to fulfill this step is to look at the report you received when you bought your home. Typically it will say that there is no known asbestos in your home. Unless you suspect that there is asbestos or you just want to be thorough, that report should suffice to satisfy this criterion.

Dale Stubbart

Author of <u>Traveling with Multiple Chemical Sensitivities</u>

Make Your Home Free of Toxic Chemicals

Separate Your Garage From Your House

If there is an attached garage, permanently separate it from your house, sealing the doorway with Denny Foil[1] or with some other odor or vapor barrier.

Alternatively, you can make your garage non–toxic and quit using it as a garage.

---

[1] Denny Foil is available at Foustco.Com. Denny Foil is sold as a vapor barrier and insulating layer.

Author of <u>Traveling with Multiple Chemical Sensitivities</u>

Make Your Home Free of Toxic Chemicals

Seal Off Toxic Areas

Seal off *toxic* areas, such as attics where there may be *toxic* insulation, with Denny Foil or with another odor or vapor barrier.

Make Your Home Free of Toxic Chemicals

Rooms to Pay the Most Attention To

Even if you removed all of the *toxic chemicals* from your bedroom in Stage One, it did you little good if you kept bringing them back into your bedroom, even if you did so unintentionally.

For that reason, the rooms that you will want to pay the most attention to during the second stage are those areas near the bedroom. If there are several bedrooms and all areas are near the

Make Your Home Free *of Toxic Chemicals*

bedrooms, then you're done! Wishful thinking!

The bedrooms should be small areas. Ideally bedrooms contain the bed and not much else. You may want to repurpose a small room as a bedroom and repurpose the bedroom as a different room. Who says that you have to keep the rooms as they were originally designated?

Keeping the bedroom small helps to keep *toxic chemicals* out of the sleeping

Make Your Home Free of *Toxic Chemicals*

area. And that is important when you're trying to help your immune system recover from *toxic chemicals* it encounters in a normal day.

Other rooms that you will want to pay special attention to during this second stage are those rooms where you want to concentrate, study, meditate, etc. It is harder to keep your mind focused when it's being inundated with *toxic chemicals*. And it can be especially hard to focus on not focusing on anything or to keep your thoughts from running wild, like you are

Make Your Home Free of Toxic Chemicals

supposed to do in some forms of meditation.

Make Your Home Free *of Toxic Chemicals*

Stage Three – Lime Green – Clean Up the Air, Water, and Light

Intro

Stage Three of our plan to rid your home of *toxic chemicals* suggests scoring 40 of 60 points from the following 6 criterion (10 points each). Completion of Stage Three includes completion of Stage Two.

Author of <u>Traveling with Multiple Chemical Sensitivities</u>

Make Your Home Free of Toxic Chemicals

At least one criterion to clean up the Air, one to clean up the Water, and one to remove toxic chemicals due to Lighting should be met. That will give you another 10 points. Yes, it is possible to score more than 60 points for this stage.

Clean Up the Air - Circulation

Install an Air Circulation System. This may be an actual system or just good cross-ventilation provided by windows and screen doors.

Make Your Home Free of Toxic Chemicals

This may have been included in your mold elimination program in Stage Two. If it was, you can score points for it also here in Stage Three.

Clean Up the Air - Filtration

Install Air Filters or bring NASA recommended House Plants into your house to filter the air. Air Filters should be changed regularly. Other alternatives for cleaning the air include Salt Crystal Lamps and Bees Wax Candles with natural wicks.

Make Your Home Free of Toxic Chemicals

Clean Up the Air – No Carpets

Carpets hold in *toxic chemicals*. Walking on carpets releases some of those toxic chemicals into the air. But after a while, those toxic chemicals settle back down into the carpet, rejoining their cousins who were buried deeper in the pile.

At least that has been my experience. And that theory is backed up by the American Lung Association – https://www.lung.org/our-initiatives/healthy-air/indoor/indoor-

Make Your Home Free of Toxic Chemicals

<u>air-pollutants/carpets.html</u> So remove all of the carpets from your house.

All of the floors in your house should be naturally sealed with Shellac or another natural sealant. Alternatively the floors can be made from wood, bamboo, stone, ceramic tile, concrete, marmoleum, or some other natural material. You may still want to seal your natural floors. These floors can then be covered with area rugs made from natural fibers if so desired.

Make Your Home Free of Toxic Chemicals

When you remove your old flooring, you will probably expose the subflooring which is below it. You may need to seal this subflooring with a natural sealer and/or Denny Foil before adding new natural flooring on top of it.

Clean Up the Air – Remove Your Shoes

Shoes can carry dirt and man-made chemicals from elsewhere into your home. They should be removed before you enter.

You'll probably want to post signs directing the removal of shoes at the

Author of <u>Traveling with Multiple Chemical Sensitivities</u>

Make Your Home Free of Toxic Chemicals

entryways of your home. The signs can designate where shoes can be left, if that's not obvious. I myself, like the signs we have from Hawaii which say, *Please Remove your Slippas,* and which show a pair of flip-flops.

Clean Up the Water - Filtration

Install a Drinking Water Filter. Most homes are on a community (or city) water systems where the water is treated before entering your home. Most community water systems use Chlorine

Author of <u>Traveling with Multiple Chemical Sensitivities</u>

Make Your Home Free
of Toxic Chemicals

to treat the water. Chlorine is a *toxic chemical*.

There are a few systems which use ultra-violet light to filter the water. But most of those use ultra-violet light in conjunction with chlorine. Using the ultra-violet light means that they can use less chlorine.

Most community water systems also use Fluoride to treat the water. Even if your community water system does not treat the water with *toxic* (in our minds) or questionable *chemicals*, the water may

Make Your Home Free of *Toxic Chemicals*

pick up other things (minerals, bacteria, etc.) on its way through the pipes to your house. Water filters should be changed regularly.

Alternatives to filtering your drinking water are well water, where the well is tested regularly; and bottled water. Bottled water in plastic bottles may run the risk of the plastic leaching phthalates and other *toxic chemicals* into the water.

You should also install shower filters. The same rules as those which apply to drinking water filters, apply to shower

Make Your Home Free of Toxic Chemicals

filters. Whatever method you choose to filter your water, you'll want to use non-toxic water for showers, baths, etc., as well as for drinking.

In the shower, *toxic chemicals* vaporize into the air. You can breathe them in through your nose or through the pores in your skin. For some, this is worse than drinking unfiltered water.

Remove Toxic Chemicals Due to Lighting

We encourage you to try and use natural lighting via the sun. You may want to change your home to increase

Author of <u>Traveling with Multiple Chemical Sensitivities</u>

Make Your Home Free of Toxic Chemicals

the natural lighting. This may include adding windows, skylights, and full spectrum lighting.

There is also fiber-optic technology which will bring the natural sunlight indoors. This fiber-optic technology is sometimes referred to as hybrid solar lighting.

For homes in areas where natural lighting is not always available, due to weather or trees or your neighbor's house, natural lighting from the sun should be supplemented by other means.

Make Your Home Free of Toxic Chemicals

Full spectrum lightbulbs are available as regular lightbulbs, CFL's, and LED's. CFL's contain mercury. This is a very small amount of mercury. The amount of mercury in a CFL is less than the amount in a watch battery, amalgam filling, or mercury thermometer. But mercury is a *toxic chemical* none-the-less.

Broken CFL's should be treated as hazardous waste. The EPA has simple recommendations for how to clean up a broken CFL – https://www.epa.gov/cfl/cleaning-broken-cfl. Philip's has pledged to

Make Your Home Free of Toxic Chemicals

remove both lead and mercury from its light bulbs.

Full Spectrum LED's are available. And LED's are mercury–free. Not only that, they use less energy.

Author of <u>Traveling with Multiple Chemical Sensitivities</u>

Make Your Home Free of Toxic Chemicals

Rooms to Pay the Most Attention To

The rooms to pay the most attention to during this stage are the bathroom, laundry room, and the entrance areas. Fragrances and other *toxic chemical* from cleansers, personal care products, and laundry detergents tend to accumulate in the bathroom and laundry room. It may take extra filtration and cleaning to remove these *toxic chemical* from those rooms.

Author of <u>Traveling with Multiple Chemical Sensitivities</u>

Make Your Home Free of Toxic Chemicals

The entryways are where most *toxic chemical* enter your house. So pay some extra attention to filtering are at the entrances.

Make Your Home Free of Toxic Chemicals

Stage Four – Living Green – Extra Air Purification

Intro

Stage Four of our plan to rid your home of *toxic chemicals* suggests scoring 45 of 70 points from the following 7 criterion (10 points each). Completion of Stage Four includes completion of the previous stages.

Make Your Home Free of Toxic Chemicals

Vacuum Cleaner

Your vacuum cleaner should contain both a HEPA (High Efficiency Particulate Air) and an ULPA (Ultra Low Particulate Air) filter. A HEPA filter is an extra fine filter. An ULPA filter is an ultra-fine filter. Vacuum cleaners with both of these filters will remove most (99.999%) of the dust, pollen, mold, bacteria, particles (even very tiny ones) from the air which passes through them.

Author of <u>Traveling with Multiple Chemical Sensitivities</u>

Make Your Home Free of Toxic Chemicals

Bedroom Air

The requirement for this criterion is to make sure that the air in the bedroom is filtered very well.

Electronics

You will also want to place extra filtration near electronics such as computers, TV's, and stereo systems. Electronics may be fire-proofed with PBDE's (Polybrominated Diphenyl Ethers). PBDE's started being phased out in 2009. Still, electronics often come laced with *toxic chemicals* which are hard to clean up. Alternatively, you can

Make Your Home Free of Toxic Chemicals

enclose these electronics away from living areas.

Initial Removal of Residual Toxic Chemicals

One method of removing residual *toxic chemicals* from the air is to leave dry black tea bags throughout your house for a month. Renew the tea bags on a weekly basis. The strewn tea bags pulls *toxic chemicals* from the air and gives your home character — what type of character, we won't say.

Make Your Home Free of *Toxic Chemicals*

Zeolite is another method of accomplishing this criterion. Zeolite clears the air by pulling the *toxic chemicals* into tiny crevices in the zeolite crystals and trapping them there.

Leaving bowls of vinegar around your house is another option if the smell of vinegar doesn't overwhelm the inhabitants.

Bowls of sea water (or at least salt water) should also do the trick.

Completely airing your house for a month, will work provided that there is

Make Your Home Free of *Toxic Chemicals*

good air circulation and provided that you're not pulling in toxic air.

On-Going Removal of Residual *Toxic Chemicals*

Continuously remove residual *toxic chemicals* from the air. The above methods should be used on an annual (or more frequent) schedule.

Other methods of continuously removing *toxic chemicals* from the air include continuously running salt crystal lamps and monthly burning of fragrance-free bees wax candles.

Make Your Home Free of Toxic Chemicals

Candles should be burned for at least 12 hours. This can be done a few hours at a time, rather than 12 hours continuously.

Radon Mitigation

Install a Passive Radon Mitigation System. A Passive Radon Mitigation System is basically a pipe which allows air to flow from the crawl space or footing below the basement to the exterior of your house above the roof.

Make Your Home Free of Toxic Chemicals

Toxic Chemical Remediation Toolkit

Ensure that you have a constant supply of toxic-remediation tools on hand. You may want to include the following in your toolkit:

- Tea Bags
- Vodka
- Baking Soda
- Vinegar
- Photocatalytic Spray
- Zeolite
- And Carbon Paper

Author of <u>Traveling with Multiple Chemical Sensitivities</u>

Make Your Home Free of Toxic Chemicals

Rooms to Pay the Most Attention To

If you have a furnace room, utility closet, basement, crawl space, and/or attic, you will want to pay the most attention to those rooms during this phase.

Author of <u>Traveling with Multiple Chemical Sensitivities</u>

Make Your Home Free of *Toxic Chemicals*

Stage Five – Avocado Green – Further Interior Remediation

Intro

Stage Five of our plan to rid your home of *toxic chemicals* suggests scoring 50 of 80 points from the following 8 criterion (10 points each). Completion of Stage Five includes completion of the

Make Your Home Free of Toxic Chemicals

previous stages. Stage Five could be called the Seal and Monitor Stage.

Seal Furniture

Seal your furniture with natural sealers and/or use furniture made with natural products. If the dressers, shelves, etc. of your home are not made with natural products, seal them with natural shellac or another natural sealant. You will want to especially seal the interiors of dressers.

Alternatively, you can line the interiors of your dressers and shelves with sheets

Make Your Home Free of Toxic Chemicals

of carbon paper or with bags of zeolite. Zeolite and carbon paper need to sit in the sun every so often to remain effective. Tea bags will also work. Just replace them when they become ineffective.

Seal Cabinets

Seal your cabinets with natural sealers and/or use cabinets made with natural products. If the cabinets are not made with natural products, seal them with natural shellac or with another natural sealant. You will want to especially seal the interiors of your cabinets.

Make Your Home Free of Toxic Chemicals

Alternatively, you can line the interiors of your cabinets with sheets of carbon paper or with bags of zeolite. Zeolite and carbon paper need to sit in the sun every so often to remain effective.

Seal Wall Cracks

Seal any cracks in the walls of your house with a non-toxic sealant to reduce exposure to *toxic chemicals* trapped in the walls. Consider mud plaster or other natural plaster for all of your walls and ceilings – use where appropriate. If you are repainting, use no-voc paints.

Make Your Home Free of Toxic Chemicals

If you did not hire a professional mold remover in Stage Two, do so now. If there is mold in our walls, remediate it before sealing them. Mold will continue to grow and spread even if it is sealed in. And the mold will eventually seep through the seal or spread beyond it.

Some people say to scrub the walls with bleach to kill the mold. But according to the professional builder website, the only way to properly remove mold is to remove whatever has mold on it. Besides, most bleach has chlorine in it.

Dale Stubbart
Author of <u>Traveling with Multiple Chemical Sensitivities</u>

Make Your Home Free of Toxic Chemicals

If possible, also remediate toxic chemicals in the walls before sealing them. The toxic chemicals will also eventually seep through the seal.

No Gas

To satisfy this criterion, replace all of your gas and propane appliances with electric ones. Shut off the gas inlets to your home permanently. Shutting them off permanently may require hiring a mechanic or calling the gas company to send one out.

Make Your Home Free of Toxic Chemicals

Remove Lead

Properly remediate any lead paint within your home. There shouldn't be any lead paint in your home in the first place. It should have been remediated before you bought it. If it wasn't you'll want to remediate it now.

The simplest method is to cover the paint with a coating that is made for this purpose.
https://www.houselogic.com/remodel/painting-lighting/lead-paint-removal/

Make Your Home Free of Toxic Chemicals

Monitor Carbon Monoxide

Meter or test carbon monoxide levels in your home. Make sure that they are at a safe level. Carbon monoxide is usually not a problem when there are no gas or propane appliances.

You may be required to install carbon monoxide monitors before you can sell your home. Even if you are not required to install them, it is still a good idea to do so.

Make Your Home Free of Toxic Chemicals

Monitor Electro-Magnetic Frequencies (EMFs)

Meter or test EMF levels in your home. Make sure that they are at a safe level. The internationally recognized safe-level for EMF's is based on the ICNIRP (International Commission on Non-Ionizing Radiation Protection) recommendations (basically 2 milligauss). You may want to use a more precautionary standard such as that of Switzerland (basically .2 milligauss).

An easy way to lower the EMF levels in your home is to place all laptops,

Make Your Home Free of Toxic Chemicals

phones, etc. into airplane mode when you don't need to connect to the internet. When you do need to connect, use an ethernet cable on your laptop.

Also use the USB cable which came with your smart phone to transfer pictures from your phone to your laptop. This will be the same cable that you plug into the power connector to charge your phone.

Make Your Home Free of Toxic Chemicals

Monitor Radon

Meter or test radon levels in your home. Make sure that they are at a safe level.

Radon tends to be a problem in certain geographic areas (due to the geology). It is often not a problem in other areas.

Radon tends to be a problem in homes with basements in these geographic areas. Some locations require new homes built in those areas to have Radon Mitigation Systems installed.

Make Your Home Free of Toxic Chemicals

Rooms to Pay the Most Attention To

Pay attention to any rooms to which you haven't paid special attention to before such as living room, kitchen, dining room, hallways, etc.

Also, if you need to pay special attention to any room in your house again, do so. If it is wanting your attention, don't ignore it.

Author of <u>Traveling with Multiple Chemical Sensitivities</u>

Make Your Home Free *of Toxic Chemicals*

Stage Six – Forest Green – Exterior Remediation

Intro

Stage Six of our plan to rid your home of *toxic chemicals* suggests scoring 20 of 40 points from the following 4 criterion (10 points each). Completion of Stage Six includes completion of the previous stages.

Make Your Home Free of *Toxic Chemicals*

You may consider Stages Six and Seven to be optional, and above and beyond the call of duty. They will help you rid the exterior of your home of *toxic chemicals*, but you live in the interior of your home. So these stages are not quite as critical to your well-being as the first five.

Create an Airing Station

An airing station is a place outside of your home where items containing or having absorbed *toxic chemicals* can be

Make Your Home Free of Toxic Chemicals

aired before they are brought into your home.

Create a Junk Mail Recycling Station

Mail comes from some other location which may not be non-toxic. Place your junk mail recycling station outside of your home. That way you can recycle junk mail rather than bringing it inside your home.

To remediate non-junk mail from its toxic chemicals, try tea bags, carbon paper, and/or seal it in plastic bags

Make Your Home Free of *Toxic Chemicals*

which have a sealing lock. I often seal it in these bags along with tea bags.

Screen the Road

Plant a screen of trees and/or bushes near the road and optionally along the driveway. Trees and bushes should be native to your region. They should need minimal amounts of water, other than what comes from rainfall.

The trees or bushes will absorb emissions from exhaust. They will also help keep exhaust out of your house. And that's a good thing because exhaust might tire you.

Dale Stubbart
Author of <u>Traveling with Multiple Chemical Sensitivities</u>

Make Your Home Free of Toxic Chemicals

No Idling

Reduce driveway idling emissions. This can be done by not idling your car to warm it up. This saves gas.

You can also move idling emissions further from your house by parking your car at the far end of your driveway. Having a non-Petroleum-fueled car (or no car at all) is another way to achieve this no-idling goal.

Diesel fumes are harder to breathe for some than gasoline fumes.

Make Your Home Free

of Toxic Chemicals

You should never leave your car unattended while it is idling. In some locations, leaving your car unattended while it is idling is a crime. Check with your local police or with your local DOT (Department of Transportation).

Author of <u>Traveling with Multiple Chemical Sensitivities</u>

Make Your Home Free of *Toxic Chemicals*

Rooms to Pay the Most Attention To

The rooms to pay attention to during this stage are any outside *rooms* that you build for your airing station or junk mail recycling station. You will want to build them out of non-toxic materials. They should also have ventilation so that the toxic fumes from what you're airing and from your junk mail don't accumulate in them.

Dale Stubbart

Author of <u>Traveling with Multiple Chemical Sensitivities</u>

Make Your Home Free *of Toxic Chemicals*

Stage Seven – Emerald Green – Further Exterior Remediation

Intro

Stage Seven of our plan to rid your home of *toxic chemicals* suggests scoring 30 of 60 points from the following 6 criterion (10 points each). Completion of Stage Seven includes completion of the previous stages.

Make Your Home Free of Toxic Chemicals

Exterior Asbestos Remediation

Properly remediate all asbestos on the outside of your home. This will probably require a permit.

It is usually far less expensive to remediate this asbestos yourself, rather than hiring a contractor. That's because the fee for a permit for asbestos removal for a contractor is usually much higher than the fee for a permit for an individual.

Make Your Home Free of Toxic Chemicals

Usually exterior asbestos is in the form of wall tiles. The wall tiles contain asbestos. However, the asbestos is usually not a problem unless it is released from the tiles if they break.

Still, it may be difficult to sell a home which has asbestos tiles. So, it is in your interest to remove them and to replace them with non-toxic walls.

Exterior Lead Paint Remediation

Properly remediate all lead paint on the exterior of your home. If you are

Author of <u>Traveling with Multiple Chemical Sensitivities</u>

Make Your Home Free of *Toxic Chemicals*

repainting, after removing the lead-based paint, use no-voc paints.

Exterior Arsenic Remediation

Remove all arsenic-treated wood. Replace it with a non-toxic alternative.

Exterior Non-Porous Paths Remediation

Replace non-porous paths such as side-walks and driveways with paths which have porous surfaces. This keeps the *toxic chemicals* in the water from standing in one place. This also helps to

Make Your Home Free of *Toxic Chemicals*

filter the *toxic chemicals*, rather than running them directly into the rainwater sewer which may eventually be returned to your home in the form of tap water.

Porous concrete is available as a replacement option for your paths. Alternatively, you can use wood chips, gravel, oyster shells, or some similar natural material to create porous paths.

Green Roof

Replace the roof of your house with one which is made of natural materials such as metal. Another way to make

Make Your Home Free of Toxic Chemicals

your roof green is to have a living roof – one which is covered with vegetation. These plants will also help to filter the air.

It is a good idea to investigate living roofs before you turn your roof into one. You will want to make sure your house will support a living roof and that it won't leak into your home.

While you are replacing the roof of your house, it is a good time to install skylights for extra natural lighting into the interior of your home.

Dale Stubbart

Author of <u>Traveling with Multiple Chemical Sensitivities</u>

Make Your Home Free of Toxic Chemicals

You may also want to make the roof of your garage green.

Filter Exterior Water

Filter your outside water. This can be done via a carbon filter on the hose. Alternatively, you can let the water sit in a bucket for a few hours before using it. Be certain to cover the bucket with a screen to keep mosquitoes from laying their eggs in it.

Other alternate methods include using well water and/or rain water. It is best to filter the rain water coming off of

Make Your Home Free of Toxic Chemicals

your roof, especially if you have asphalt tiles and tar paper on your roof.

Flow forms are another alternative for filtering water. These geometric shapes filter the water the same way as nature does as the water flows through them.

Filtration gardens are yet another alternative. Filtration gardens are also called rain gardens.

Make Your Home Free of Toxic Chemicals

Rooms to Pay the Most Attention To

This stage is about remediating the outside of your home. During the first five stages you paid special attention to all of the rooms in your house. Now it is time to pay special attention to your garage, shed, and other outbuildings.

If you have an outhouse, you probably already paid special attention to it during Stage Two when you paid special attention to your bathroom. If your outhouse is a chemical toilet, make sure

Make Your Home Free of Toxic Chemicals

it uses the least-toxic chemicals available.

Dale Stubbart
Author of <u>Traveling with Multiple Chemical Sensitivities</u>

Make Your Home Free
of Toxic Chemicals

The Simpler Plan

This is the simpler plan to rid your home of toxic chemicals. This plan takes the most important criterion from the stages of the comprehensive plan. The comprehensive plan is the plan which was outlined in the previous chapters of this book.

The Simpler Plan includes Stage One:
- Remove All Air Fresheners
- Switch to Natural Laundry Products

Author of <u>Traveling with Multiple Chemical Sensitivities</u>

Make Your Home Free of Toxic Chemicals

- Switch to Natural, Non–Toxic Personal Care Products
- Smoking is Not Allowed

You'll also want to pay special attention to your bedroom as in Stage One.

From Stage Two, you will want to hire a Professional Mold Inspector. Also from Stage Two, seal off any toxic areas. This may include sealing off your garage from your house.

Make Your Home Free of Toxic Chemicals

From Stage Three, filter your air and water. You will also want to get rid of your carpets.

From Stage Four, create your own Toxic Chemical Remediation Toolkit.

From Stage Five, replace your gas appliances with electric ones.

From Stage Six, no-idling in your driveway if you have a diesel vehicle. If you do have a diesel vehicle, you should seriously consider trading it on a non-

Make Your Home Free of Toxic Chemicals

diesel vehicle, especially if it's an older vehicle. I don't know if you're more sensitive to diesel than gasoline; but everybody I know who is sensitive to either fumes, is more sensitive to diesel.

I didn't include any criterion from Stage Seven in this Simpler Plan.

This simpler plan includes about a dozen criteria. You should perform all of them. There is no 8 out of 12 option in this plan.

Author of <u>Traveling with Multiple Chemical Sensitivities</u>

Make Your Home Free of Toxic Chemicals

If you opt for this simpler plan, when you finish it, go back and check the steps which you skipped in the comprehensive plan to see if you are wanting to perform any of them.

Make Your Home Free of Toxic Chemicals

About the Author & His Wife

The author and his wife were married in 1984. His wife thought that she was just running a little low on energy and that she would recover soon enough. She thought that she just needed a little rest.

Less than a year later, she came home with the diagnosis that she was *allergic to everything man-made*. What we knew at that point was that she was allergic to everything made from

Author of <u>Traveling with Multiple Chemical Sensitivities</u>

Make Your Home Free of Toxic Chemicals

petroleum, especially diesel and new asphalt. She was also allergic to sulfur.

We were renting an apartment in a suburb of Minneapolis at the time. There was not a lot of refurbishing we could do, since we didn't own our home.

We quit using the gas stove and bought a hot-plate instead. We had a microwave at the time which served as an oven.

When my wife discovered that she was allergic to fragrance, nobody understood. And most were not willing

Author of <u>Traveling with Multiple Chemical Sensivities</u>

Make Your Home Free of Toxic Chemicals

to leave off their fragrance when they were around her.

Our Christmas Tree was made out of green paper-board.

It would just be a matter of time. It would just be a matter of finding the right doctors.

One doctor had my wife take the MMPI – Minnesota Multiphasic Personality Inventory. The MMPI is a test to see if you need psychological help. That doctor didn't realize that this disease was body-based rather than brain-based. My wife is definitely sane.

Dale Stubbart

Author of <u>Traveling with Multiple Chemical Sensitivities</u>

Make Your Home Free of Toxic Chemicals

Later we learned that the hypothalamus (part of the brain) can keep the response programs running. This means that even when toxic chemicals are not driving you crazy, your body can react as though they are.

That does not mean that toxic chemicals are not responsible for your low energy and face pain. It just means that they may not be responsible for all of it. And they together with stress are probably what got your hypothalamus all worked up in the first place.

Make Your Home Free of Toxic Chemicals

Next we moved to a suburb of Columbus, Ohio. My idea. A positively bad idea.

Note: If your spouse has Multiple Chemical Sensitivities (MCS) do not move, unless you are moving into a house where you can better control which chemicals are free to come and go.

We moved into an apartment again. We had a little more control over our environment, but not much. We bought an air filter to help clear the air in the apartment.

Dale Stubbart

Author of <u>Traveling with Multiple Chemical Sensitivities</u>

Make Your Home Free of Toxic Chemicals

My wife became pretty much house-bound. She pretty much only went out to walk in the park, shop for groceries, visit my family, and go to church.

Church was the worst for breathing. So I hooked a length of dryer vent to the air filter and we took that with us. My wife put her head into the other end of the dryer vent so that she could breathe. It would have been much simpler to just stop going to church. But we didn't know that was an option.

Later we found I Can Breathe masks. These worked almost as good as the

Author of <u>Traveling with Multiple Chemical Sensivities</u>

Make Your Home Free of Toxic Chemicals

modified air filter. And they looked much nicer.

My wife kept saying that she just needed some sun. So I got the bright idea that we should move to Arizona. We talked about it. And I thought that we had agreed to do so.

Note: If your spouse has MCS, do not move her away from her friends. She needs all of the support she can get.

We moved into an apartment in Tucson, because I still didn't have a clue about what all it would take to create a

Make Your Home Free of Toxic Chemicals

safe environment. We thought we just needed to change the products that we used. We did move into a house in Tucson later. But that was for a different reason.

The floor tile in the house that we moved into was a problem. So I removed it. Carpets went. We sealed cabinets. Things were a little better.

However, when you know that you have respiratory problems due to fouled air, and you see the brown line of pollution, sand, and dust on the mountains every night; you start to

Make Your Home Free of Toxic Chemicals

think that it's time to move. So my wife suggested that we move.

It probably took me a long time to hear her. But when I finally did, I had no objection.

We moved to a house in the mountains of Colorado. At 7700 ft, there's lots of fresh air.

I was telecommuting, so I did the grocery shopping. I love to grocery shop anyway, and I could make time during the day to do that. That was a win-win.

Dale Stubbart

Author of <u>Traveling with Multiple Chemical Sensitivities</u>

Make Your Home Free of Toxic Chemicals

We no longer went to church – we were taking a hiatus from that activity. My wife made some friends that she visited from time to time. And mostly she stayed at home.

Our house this time was a manufactured home. We knew better than to move into a manufactured home – too much formaldehyde. But this was not your typical manufactured home. We didn't even know that it was manufactured.

Since we owned this home, we were able to make lots of modifications. However, the flooring couldn't be

Author of <u>Traveling with Multiple Chemical Sensitivities</u>

Make Your Home Free of Toxic Chemicals

removed – at least not easily. So, we left it alone.

Because we lived a long way from town, we started ordering items over the internet – even though the internet was fairly new then and you couldn't order much. I started developing my chemical sensitivity resource website – https://www.princesstigerlily.com/mcs.

While living here, I wrote a book of humor while living with MCS – <u>What would Terry Do?</u>

Dale Stubbart   Page **134** of **140**
Author of <u>Traveling with Multiple Chemical Sensitivities</u>

Make Your Home Free of Toxic Chemicals

Then I ran out of work and we needed to move near my new job. My wife looked at air pollution maps and decided that it would be better to live in Thurston County Washington rather than in Pierce County where the job was.

That was fine. I hadn't discovered that I really didn't like to drive yet.

I found a nice area in Thurston County, outside of Olympia that was near the ocean. It would be good for both of us to breathe that ocean air.

Dale Stubbart   Page **135** of **140**
Author of <u>Traveling with Multiple Chemical Sensitivities</u>

Make Your Home Free of Toxic Chemicals

There was a house for sale – just our size. I walked in with the realtor. I noticed the plug-in air freshener and walked right back out. There was no way we were going to be able to live there, not when they'd perfumed it like that.

A few weeks later, another house came up for sale on the same street. This one was twice as large. But it was selling for the same price. There were no plug-in air fresheners in this one. And it looked fairly safe – chemical-wise.

Dale Stubbart

Author of <u>Traveling with Multiple Chemical Sensitivities</u>

Make Your Home Free of Toxic Chemicals

For the next year, my wife lived in Colorado while I worked in Washington and spent my evenings and weekends tearing out carpeting and working with contractors to get the house ready for her to move in.

We've lived here for 15 years now. We still make mistakes (at least I do) when it comes to toxic chemicals. Life has gotten easier,. But it's never a breeze.

The hardest part now is that I travel for work and pick up a lot of toxic chemicals on my trips. If I didn't travel for

Dale Stubbart

Author of <u>Traveling with Multiple Chemical Sensitivities</u>

Make Your Home Free of Toxic Chemicals

work, I would probably still pick up chemicals from work. But at least I wouldn't pick up chemicals from my travels.

But that's the life we have. So we learn how to make it work. And traveling, led me to write <u>Traveling with Multiple Chemical Sensitivities</u>.

The other thing that is really bad is that people use really smelly toxic chemicals in their laundry. And that's a problem when we go for walks.

Dale Stubbart   Page **138** of **140**
Author of <u>Traveling with Multiple Chemical Sensitivities</u>

Make Your Home Free of Toxic Chemicals

Since I don't have to move for work – I just travel to wherever the contract is; you would think that we would stay put. However, something is drawing us to Hawaii. Partly it's better air and more sea breeze. Partly it's the warmth and the whales. Partly it's the culture.

Whatever it is, it's strong enough that we're both willing to move once more and figure out how to deal with toxic chemicals, living in a new environment.

Mostly, we're willing to make this move because Hawaii feels like home. We'll also have this book – Make Your

Author of Traveling with Multiple Chemical Sensitivities

Make Your Home Free of Toxic Chemicals

Home Free of Toxic Chemicals – as a reference whether we build a new house or move into an existing one.

Dale Stubbart   Page **140** of **140**
Author of <u>Traveling with Multiple Chemical Sensitivities</u>

www.ingramcontent.com/pod-product-compliance
Lightning Source LLC
Chambersburg PA
CBHW012253240726
48655CB00009B/3300